How to Have Natural Cholesterol I

the best book on essentials on how to lower bad LDL & boost good HDL via foods/diet, medications, exercise & knowing cholesterol myths for clarity

Jessica Caplain

ISBN-13:
978-1978343962

ISBN-10:
1978343965

No part of this book may be reproduced or transmitted in any form whatsoever, electronic, or mechanical, including photocopying, recording, or by any informational storage or retrieval system without express permission from the author

Copyright © 2017 JNR Publishing Group

All rights reserved

Chapter 1: Getting to know cholesterol 4
How much do you know about cholesterol? 4
What are low-density and high-density lipoproteins? 5
Your liver and cholesterol 5
Is there such a thing as good cholesterol? 6
Is bad cholesterol really bad? 7
Reasons why you need cholesterol in your body 8
Serious health conditions associated with high cholesterol levels 9
Assessing your risks 10
Knowing the numbers 11
Other risk factors to note 12
Physical tests to determine cholesterol levels 15
Chapter 2: Eat and live your way to better health 18
How fit should you be? 18
Making lifestyle changes: it's easier than you think 21
Count the calories 21
Make sure you get adequate vitamins and minerals 21
Come up with a scrumptious menu 22
Stay positive and proactive 23
Sweat it out! 23
Calories and exercise 24
How hard should you be exercising? 24
Kickstarting your road to better health and fitness 26
What makes a good fitness program? 29
Ditching your vices for longer life 29
Chapter 3: Knowing your partners in fighting cholesterol 34
What you should know about supplements 34
Essential vitamins and nutrients for lowering cholesterol 35
Prescription medications and their side effects 37
Your Top 10 go-to websites for tips 42
Chapter 4: Myth busters 47
Chapter 5: Food is life 53

Chapter 1: Getting to know cholesterol

Heart disease is one of the top killers in the world. In the United States alone, it comes first place, ahead of all types of cancer and diseases. The most common form of heart disease is heart attack, and one famous risk factor is high cholesterol.

Hundreds of studies have already shown the negative impact of high cholesterol, particularly the bad one, on a person's heart and overall health. The good news is that researchers have also founds ways to reduce your risk, and live a longer and happier life.

How much do you know about cholesterol?

It is true that you acquire cholesterol from the food you eat, but this is not the sole source. In fact, most of the cholesterol found in your body is produced by your liver. This organ uses fat, protein, and carbohydrates from food in order to create about 1 gram of cholesterol a day.

The cholesterol travels through your bloodstream in the form of lipoproteins. The fatty substances in these particles include triglycerides and cholesterol. The proteins combine with fat to create lipoproteins called apolipoproteins.

Lipoproteins undergo five phases as they change into the particles that bring cholesterol around the body:

> Chylomicrons

> Very low density lipoproteins or VLDLs

> Intermediate density lipoproteins or IDLs

> Low density lipoproteins or LDLs

> High density lipoproteins or HDLs

What are low-density and high-density lipoproteins?
Density refers to the weight of the lipoprotein, and protein weighs more than fat. Lipoproteins that contain less protein than fat are called low-density lipoproteins or LDLs, which are bad particles as they carry cholesterol to the arteries. The lipoproteins that contain more protein than fat are called high-density lipoproteins or HDLs, which are the good guys as they get cholesterol out of your system.

Your liver and cholesterol
The liver is high in cholesterol and fat. It gathers fat fragments from your blood, and utilize them to produce new fat and cholesterol that your body can use to form tissue and do other physiological tasks.

Once the chylomicron reaches the liver, it will gather fat particles and transform into the biggest form of lipoprotein, the very low-density lipoprotein or VLDL. Your liver will then send the VLDL into your body. As the VLDL travels around you, it will drop some fat, pick up cholesterol, and transform into the smaller and heavier intermediate low density lipoprotein or IDL, and then change into a slightly smaller and heavier low density lipoprotein or LDL.

The last phase happens when the LDL has released so much cholesterol and fat into the body that it is now mostly protein. This is the high density lipoprotein or HDL. The primary protein in VLDL, IDL, and LDL are part of the apolipoprotein class called the apoB. The HDLs, on the other hand, belong to apoA. Other less prominent apos are referred to as apoC and apoE.

You may have already heard about the apoA blood test. This test can tell you whether you have a high level of apoA, which also indicates how much HDLs or good cholesterol you have in the body.

Is there such a thing as good cholesterol?
HDLs deserve the name good cholesterol because these particles do not carry cholesterol into your heart. They are so dense and compact that they

cannot squeeze their way through your arteries, which is why they move away and out of your system, along with the rest of your waste.

You can consider HDL as scavengers that take out cholesterol from your heart. Having plenty of HDLs in your body reduces your risk of heart disease, regardless of your total cholesterol level. Studies have shown that people who increase their HDLs by living an active and healthy lifestyle reduce the number of cholesterol in their arteries, while removing plaque around the heart.

Is bad cholesterol really bad?
Not all LDLs are bad. In fact, there were researchers who dismissed the idea that people who were able to reach old age with high LDL levels and without any heart issues are just plain lucky.

In 2003, a group of scientists at New York City's Albert Einstein College of Medicine, along with researchers from Tufts University, University of Maryland, Boston University, and Roche Molecular Systems, conducted several tests on senior citizens and their kids and grandkids. They also ran the same tests on non-blood relatives, including their children's wives and husbands.

The team concluded that LDL levels do not predict a person's risk of heart disease, but the size of their LDLs. It means having plenty of small LDLs may increase your heart attack risk, even if your overall cholesterol is low. Pretty interesting, right?

Reasons why you need cholesterol in your body
Your body needs cholesterol, and here are the reasons why:

> It contributes in the developing cells of a growing fetus. It stimulates certain genes that direct embryonic cells to form the body parts. There have been reports about babies being born with birth defect because the fetuses failed to produce cholesterol during development. To help prevent this, pregnant women are advised not to take cholesterol-reducing medications.

> It helps protect cells in the body. Majority of the cholesterol in your body can be found in your cell membranes to help keep them strong and flexible.

> It comprises a large portion of the brain. Up to 12 percent of your brain is made of fat, which includes cholesterol. Your brain cells cannot send the messages to the rest of your body without cholesterol.

> It plays a role in maintaining hormonal balance. Cholesterol is a compound called sterol, which is made of oxygen and hydrogen atoms. Your body needs to synthesize other sterols, including cortisol, testosterone, and the male sex hormone.

> It is used to make bile. Without it, your body will not be able to make bile. As a result, you will not be able to absorb fat, which is crucial in the making of fatty tissue that protects your insides.

> It is a building block for vitamin D.

Serious health conditions associated with high cholesterol levels
As you have learned earlier, cholesterol plays an important role in protecting your cells, keeping your brain in top shape, helping your body make hormones and vitamins, and the list goes on. Under certain situations however, it can block your arteries and cause a heart attack.

Below are the negative effects of cholesterol to your body:

> It may harm your heart

LDLs are more commonly found in the body than HDLs. They can easily squeeze themselves within the walls of the heart, bringing cholesterol along. Once inside, these particles may get caught up on a lot of stuff in the artery wall and snag other particles.

This effect creates deposits called the plaque that, in time, may block the blood flowing through the blood vessels. A piece of the plaque may also break off, and cause a blood clot formation that may block the artery. These two possibilities can result to a heart attack. This is also why cardiologists, or the heart doctors, assume that having more cholesterol in the bloodstream will raise your risk for heart attack.

> It may clog up your brain

Having high cholesterol levels may also raise your risk of plaque build-up in the cranial artery. It can block the blood flowing through the cranial artery and into your brain, causing a stroke. It also means that taking preventing measures for your heart will also benefit your brain.

> It can build gallstones in your gallbladder

Cholesterol plays a significant role in bile formation, which is its good side. The bad side, however, is its contribution in the build-up of gallstones. These are rock-like lumps that develop when there are changes in the fat percentages in the bile, so the cholesterol clumps up in your gallbladder or the path leading to your intestines. About 80-95 percent of gallstones are made of cholesterol, while the rest are made of calcium.

Assessing your risks
The health risk factors generally fall into one of the three categories:

> Factors that you cannot control, such as your genes.

> Factors that you can control by taking cholesterol-lowering medications.

> Factors whose effects you cannot completely eliminate, but can lessen. You can change your lifestyle by losing weight, eating healthy, ditching vices, and exercising regularly.

High cholesterol is a risk factor for heart disease, but you have an important role to play in controlling your risks – particularly those you can manage.

Knowing the numbers
It is important to know how much cholesterol you have before deciding what to do about it. Set an appointment with your doctor, and take the necessary tests to have your health assessed. Your doctor will probably take a blood sample first before recommending other tests.

Your blood test results will show a number with "mg/dL" beside it. What does it mean? It refers to the number of milligrams of total cholesterol in every decilitre of blood. However, it does not show the figures for your low-density lipoproteins and high-density lipoproteins. The results might scare you, especially if it reflects high total cholesterol, so let the doctor provide a complete report before you panic.

In 2001, the National Cholesterol Education Program (NCEP) released a report, which stated that:

> A total cholesterol higher than 240 mg/dL is deemed "high risk" for heart disease

> A total cholesterol between 200 and 239 mg/dL puts a person at "moderate risk" for heart disease.

> A total cholesterol below 200 mg/dL is considered "desirable."

The risk of heart attack is highest for males with HDLs below 37mg/dL, and females below 47mg/dL. The risk is lowest among males with HDLs higher than 53mg/dL, and females higher than 60mg/dL.

Other risk factors to note
Millions of Americans have total cholesterol levels higher than 200mg/dL, according to the American Heart Association, placing them into the borderline high group. What are the important risk factors to note? Read on.

> Age and gender

Men in the under 50 age group are more likely to have high cholesterol levels. After hitting 50, women will edge into the lead. The blood vessels of women are more elastic than the men's. This is why women enjoy a bit more protection than men against blood clots that may clog the blood vessels and cause a heart attack.

Pregnancy reduces a woman's good cholesterol levels, but a study conducted at Kaiser Permanente in California revealed that nursing newborns for more than three months slows down the decline of HDL levels.

A child's total cholesterol level slowly increases from age two to ten, and then starts to rise and drop in a gender-related pattern. Darwin R. Labarthe, a researcher from the University of Texas (Houston), said a girl's total cholesterol level will likely peak around the age of nine, and around 16 for boys. However, a girl's cholesterol will go down for some time around age 16, and around 17 for boys.

All adults must be tested at least once to have a baseline reading for cholesterol. The American Heart Association suggests having children older than two years old with a family history of coronary artery disease tested for cholesterol.

> Family history

Your family history will say a lot about your future. If your first-degree relatives (father, mother, siblings) have high cholesterol, then you may have it, too. If any of the men in your family have had a heart attack below the age of 55, or any of the women have had it before turning 65, then you need to watch your health. All things being relative, however, the cholesterol levels of your relatives may not mirror yours.

> Ethnicity

The cholesterol figures on ethnic groups in the United States are incomplete. Many statistical data, however, exist for non-Hispanic Whites, non-Hispanic Blacks, and Mexican Americans. Meanwhile, scattered data are available for Native Americans, but there is nothing for other ethnic groups. Given this wide variety of people in the U.S., it is difficult to know which ethnic groups are at the highest risk of high cholesterol.

> Other medical conditions

Some health conditions will either affect your risk of high cholesterol or boost the negative effects of cholesterol. If you have one of the following conditions, then you might already know about those risks.

> Hypertension – The normal blood pressure varies when you have cholesterol issues.

> Diabetes – Diabetic patients often have high cholesterol levels, which is why they are advised to live a healthy lifestyle and take their medications.

> Lifestyle – There are health hazards when it comes to vices and inactivity. You can reduce your risk of high cholesterol.

> Obesity – Carrying excess pounds will increase your cholesterol level. Losing the unnecessary weight can significantly lower your cholesterol. In fact, dropping as few as five pounds can make a huge difference on your health.

> Previous heart attack – If you have had a heart attack in the past, then your doctor may have already prescribed a cholesterol-reducing medication.

Physical tests to determine cholesterol levels
The following are the recommended physical tests to see whether your arteries are still in top condition:

> Stress tests

Your doctor will stick electrodes on several parts of your body, particularly your upper torso. He or she will read the results as you use the treadmill or the stationary bike. There are times when a simple stress test gives false positives (showing that you have heart disease when you really do not) or false negatives (saying you are risk-free when you are at high risk).

For more accurate readings, your doctor will use a sestamibi stress test or thallium stress test. These two tests start with an injection that has radioactive sestamibi or thallium. Your doctor will give you the shot, and then ask you to wait for a few hours to let the substance reach your blood vessels.

Electrodes will be placed on various parts of your upper torso, and you will be asked to step on the treadmill or hop on the stationary bike. Your doctor will check your blood flow through those electrodes. Next, you will be asked to lie on a table as the X-ray machine detects the substance in your body. The trouble spots will become clearly visible at this point.

> Angiogram

An angiogram is only for people who are showing signs of an imminent heart attack. Your doctor, a radiologist or cardiologist, will insert a tiny tube called a catheter into your artery. This is where the dye will flow to reach your bloodstream, which can be seen (in real time) through the X-ray monitor.

If the dye suddenly stops or slows down, then it may mean that there is a narrowed or clogged area. In this case, your doctor may perform angioplasty immediately to clear the blood vessels. The doctor may insert a stent, which is a tiny spring, into the artery to keep it open. A coronary bypass surgery may be necessary when you have multiple clogged arteries or when an angioplasty cannot be done.

> Electron-beam-computed Tomography (ECBT)

Also known as the ultrafast CAT scan, the ECBT is an injection-free scan that produces snapshots of your heart, coronary arteries, and lunges to detect calcium deposits. This test is about seven times faster than the regular CAT scan, and usually only takes around five minutes to conduct.

It is the ideal medical examination to determine whether you have heart disease, especially when you need the results right away. However, the ECBT is expensive, ranging from $300 to $500. Some insurance companies do not cover such test because they have not yet considered it as basic medicine.

If you want to know how your heart is doing, you might want to see your doctor and consider having one of these tests. It will not only prepare you for the worst case scenario, but it will also allow you to reassess your lifestyle so you can live longer.

Chapter 2: Eat and live your way to better health

You can never really tell whether a person is fit or overweight just by looking at their appearance. It is not a reliable method for knowing an individual's overall health and fitness because it will depend on who is looking and what cultural standards are being applied. In order to see your fitness level accurately, you will need something more scientific.

How fit should you be?

Modern nutrition provides reasonable options to help you determine when one is overweight, including:

> Body shape

Healthy people have some body fat. Generally, women have more body fat than men, while the latter have more muscle tissue than the former. Where the accumulated fat is stored in the body is gender-related: men are more likely to have excess fat around the mid-section (abdomen), while women often complain about having flabs around their butt, hips, and thighs.

People who are mid-section heavy are called apple-shaped, while those who are bottom-heavy are referred to as pear-shaped. In order to know your body shape, here are simple steps that you can follow:

> Get a tape measure and run it around your waist

> Measure your hips

> Take the waist measurement and divide it by the hip measurement

For example: Your waist measures 29 inches, and your hips show 39 inches. You will get a waist-to-hip ratio of 0.74.

You may be at higher risk of weight-related health issues if your waist-to-hip ratio is more than 0.8 (for women) or 0.95 (for men). These are apple shape numbers.

> Weight charts

The weight charts have changed through the years, but they have been forgiving and friendly. In 1990, the dietary guidelines for Americans showed that women weigh less than men of the same age and height because the former have smaller frames than the latter. In 2005, however, all weight charts were tossed out in favor of the Body Mass Index (BMI) chart.

> Body composition

BMI is the measurement of weight relative to height to predict a person's risk for weight-related health issues, like diabetes and heart disease. The unisex chart will show you that the higher the number, the higher the risk.

The original equation used kilograms and meters for weight and height, respectively, where: BMI = W/H2. If you want to compute using pounds and inches, then you can compute for your BMI this way: BMI = W/H2*705.

Based on the death and health statistics released by the World Health Organization, and the National Center for Health Statistics, the BMI categories are as follows:

> Underweight: BMI lower than 18.5.

> Normal: 18.5 to 24.9. (minimal risk)

> Overweight: 25 to 29.9. (moderate risk)

> Obese: 30 to 39.9. (High risk)

> Extremely obese: Over 40. (highest risk)

BMI is a good health predictor for men and women, particularly between 19 and 70 years old, but it is not for everyone. It is no longer reliable for the following cases:

> Pregnant or nursing women

> People who are very short or very tall

> Professional athletes or body builders

Making lifestyle changes: it's easier than you think

Changing your lifestyle to lower your cholesterol levels, and improving your overall health is not as difficult as you think. The road to health and fitness is simple and sensible, in fact. Once you have decided to take this path, the following tips will be extremely useful along the way:

Count the calories

A healthy weight loss routine does not include starvation. Take note of this guideline to help you better manage your calorie intake:

> Women need at least 1,200 calories a day, with a top limit of 1,500 calories.

> Men need at least 1,500 calories a day, with a top limit of 1,800 calories.

You probably noticed that men get to eat more every day than women. This is because a man's body has more muscle tissue than a woman's body. This muscle tissue is active and burns calories, which is why men need around 10 percent more calories daily, even as they try to lose weight.

Make sure you get adequate vitamins and minerals

Your weight loss meal plan should contain all the essential nutrients. A good guide to your daily vitamins and minerals is the ingredients label on a

nt brand. Many people fall victim to silly food plans,
t promise to take off 30 pounds in just 30 days.

The American Society of Bariatric Physicians,

> To lose one pound of body weight, you need to cut out 3,500 calories every day

> To drop 30 pounds in a month, you must take out a total of 105,000 calories.

> If you usually consume 2,800 calories a day, then you only need to consume 84,000 calories in 30 days.

> If you will starve yourself for 30 days, then you will still need to cut another 21,000 calories to hit the 105,000-calorie mark.

Are you feeling hungry now? Ditch the pound-a-day promises. The healthy way to lose weight is to slowly drop five pounds in 30 days, meaning you only need to cut 17,500 calories. Divide this by 30, and you will get 580 calories deficit each day. This is a realistic and healthy goal.

Come up with a scrumptious menu
A healthy meal plan can still be satiating. Food variety is crucial because you can only get the needed vitamins and minerals from various sources.

Besides, if your menu tastes good, then sticking to a healthy meal plan becomes less of a chore. Do yourself a favor and avoid fad diets.

Stay positive and proactive
Most people who want to lose weight often end up gaining them back within three years. The only way to successfully keep the pounds off is to change your mindset. Your goal should be a life-long healthy mind and body.

Remember: never rely on the scale alone

The truth is that people gain more weight as they age, but many of them manage to remain healthy and fit anyway. The older folks are still alive today because their overall health is so impressive that weight has become irrelevant. It is also important to understand that everyone is different, with unique sets of genes. Never try to make them fit into a set of strict categories.

Sweat it out!
Regular exercise is an important part of living a healthy lifestyle. In fact, the 2005 Dietary Guidelines for Americans mentioned "Physical Activity" whenever possible. The American Heart Association also agreed that exercise can reduce your cholesterol levels, boost your HDLs (the good guys), and lower down your LDLs (the bad ones).

Exercise is basically moving. There are two ways to estimate the effectiveness of an exercise: by counting the calories burned and by counting your heart rate as you do perform the movement.

Calories and exercise

The more calories you consume as you exercise, the harder you are working. To gauge your physical fitness level, here is a quick guide:

> Very light activity (80-100 calories-per-hour). Examples: Painting pictures, typing, driving, sewing, cooking, ironing, playing a musical instrument, playing cards

> Light (110-160 calories-per-hour). Examples: House cleaning, walking on a level surface at 2.5-3.0mph, golf, child care

> Moderate (170-240 calories-per-hour). Examples: Weeding, walking 3.5-4.0mph, dancing, bicycling

> Heavy (250-350 calories-per-hour). Examples: Carrying items uphill, climbing, heavy digging, football, basketball, soccer

How hard should you be exercising?

Aerobic literally means "with air." Performing aerobic exercises will force your body to use oxygen, and challenge your heart to pump more and your lungs to function double-time. Most exercises that make you use big muscle groups (legs, chest, back) are aerobic. Running, walking, swimming, climbing, and biking, are examples of aerobic exercises.

So, how fast should your heart be beating during workout? Take a pen and a piece of paper, and follow these steps to know your target heart rate range during exercise:

> Subtract your age from 220. This will be your estimated maximum heart rate.

> Divide your estimated max. heart rate by 2 to get the low point for your target range.

> Multiply the estimated max. Heart rate by 0.85 to obtain the top boundary for your target rate.

You must reach – and maintain – your target range for at least 30 minutes in order to burn fat and get results. It is advisable to do aerobic exercises at least three times a week, but make sure to get your doctor's approval first.

Exercising regularly will make your heart healthy, but did you know that it will also help improve your cholesterol profile? It's time to get moving, soldier!

The same exercise heart-strengthening regimen will

> Reduce your total cholesterol levels

> Reduce your LDLs or the bad cholesterol

> Increase your HDLs or the good cholesterol

The American Society of Bariatric Physicians sees regular exercise as a predictor for long-term healthy weight management. While you can lose weight just by cutting calories, this organization believes that you will drop the pounds faster and keep them off longer when you exercise regularly. Furthermore, exercising can also improve your body shape, which is something nearly everyone is so desperate to achieve.

Important: The first step to a healthy exercise regimen is to see your doctor for a basic body check. A stress test may even be recommended to make sure that your body is ready to exercise.

Kickstarting your road to better health and fitness
Your exercise program should make you feel great, both inside and out. If you choose a routine that is too strenuous, then you might quit in the

middle of the program. Your goal is to rev up your body and improve your overall health.

Here are a few helpful tips:

> Have realistic expectations.

There is a popular saying, "Rome wasn't built in a day." It means working your way to a fit and healthy body will not happen instantly. Start small. If you have been sedentary for many years, then you should not expect to become athletic in just a few days or weeks. Give yourself ample time to adapt to the changes.

> Have a rest day or two

Rest days are as important as your workout days. You can exercise up to six days a week, but make sure to allot one day to let your body recharge and repair damaged muscles. When you workout, your muscles suffer from micro tears, but do not be frightened by this as it is part of the process. You should, however, allow your body to rest and recover to repair those torn muscles and give room for improvements.

> Have a cheat day

A healthy lifestyle is encouraged, but you can combat plateau by giving yourself a cheat day. While you can stuff yourself with pancakes or burgers during cheat day, a good reward can be a new set of clothes or staying in bed all day. You can indulge in food rewards, but make sure to do it less often.

> Choose activities you like

Choose activities that are fun. Aim to find a physical activity that you will enjoy. It should also fit your schedule. If you choose a routine that you hate, then chances are you will not make it past the first week.

> Stick to the schedule

Make sure to perform moderate-intensity exercises for at least 30 minutes a day, five to six days a week. If you have a busy schedule, then try to workout at least three days per week and avoid skipping a session as much as you can.

> Listen to your body

The saying, "no pain, no gain," is already outdated. Experiencing too much pain means injury, and injury is bad for you. It is normal to feel uncomfortable during exercise, but it should not leave you hobbling.

What makes a good fitness program?
Your program should:

> Fit into your schedule, instead of forcing you to completely turnaround your life to accommodate it

> Make you feel great afterwards

> Match your current fitness level

> Match your budget

If you are signing up for a gym membership, then you have to make sure that the instructor has all the credentials needed. Your trainer should have a four-year college degree in sports science, physical therapy, or any related field.

Ditching your vices for longer life
Your health is negatively affected not only by the food you eat, but also by your vices. Getting rid of them in your life will make remarkable improvements in your overall health. If you have been drinking, smoking, and doing drugs then you want to reassess your lifestyle and make some healthy changes.

> Smoking

Smoking will:

> Increase the presence of carbon monoxide in your blood and reduce your body's oxygen levels.

> Injure the blood vessel lining

> Constrict the arteries that may have been narrowed by plaque

> Increase your risk of hypertension

> Lower the amount of oxygen-carrying blood to your tissues

> Increase the probability of blood clot

> Raise your risk of sudden cardiac arrest

> Raise your risk of cancer

Smoking has also been linked to increased cholesterol levels. It will decrease your good cholesterol levels, boost the plaque build-up on your blood vessels, restrict blood flow, raise your triglyceride level, and double your risk of heart attack. Secondhand smoke is also something that you will want to avoid, because inhaling other people's cigar will cause damage to your health.

When you finally decide to quit, there are three ways to do it:

> Just quit

> Quit with the help of prescribed medications

> Quit by undergoing behaviour-changing program

A person's risk of smoking-related coronary artery disease increases based on the number of cigarettes smoked per day. Furthermore,

> People who quit smoking reduce their CAD risk by half

> People who quit after a heart attack or undergoing coronary artery bypass procedure reduce their risk of early death

> People who quit reduces their likelihood of illness as well as risk of death

> Alcohol

Alcoholic beverages are one of mankind's simple pleasures. Moderate drinking was found to be beneficial to the heart, but excessive consumption is already hazardous to your health. The 2005 Dietary Guidelines for Americans revealed the following effects of moderate drinking:

> Reduces total cholesterol

> Increases good cholesterol levels

> Relaxes the muscles

> Helps lower blood pressure

As soon as you take a sip of that alcoholic beverage,

> Small amounts will head into your bloodstream. The process is so fast that the alcohol will reach your brain in just seconds.

> Most of it will go to your organs

> It will relax the heart muscles, meaning it will pump out less blood for a while and reduce your risk of stroke and heart attack due to blood clotting.

> The contractions will return to normal, but the blood vessels may stay relaxed and your blood pressure may remain lowered for as long as 30 minutes.

The positive effects of moderate drinking is nearly immediate, but how do you determine the ideal amount of alcohol you should be taking? According to the Dietary Guidelines, one drink a day for women, and two drinks per day for men.

The recommended amount is different for men and women because of the enzymes released by the body to metabolize the alcohol. The average woman produces less alcohol-metabolizing enzyme than the average man. This is why most women get tipsy much faster than men.

The American Heart Association defined one drink as:

> 5oz of wine

> 12oz of the regular beer

> 1.5oz of 80-proof distilled spirits

> 1oz of 100-proof distilled spirits

Excessive alcohol drinking may cause:

> Birth defects

> Cancer

> Allergic reaction to the sulful compounds found in some wines – this can be life-threatening

> Body pains the next day (stomach pains, dehydration, headache, muscle pain)

> Drug interactions

There is no 100 percent alcohol. It is always mixed with water, and possibly some food residue from where it was made.

In addition, alcohol does not contain any nutrients other than energy (about seven calories per gram). This means distilled spirits, like whiskey, have only calories to offer. Fermented beverages (wine, beer, cider, etc) have some residue from the food they were made. They may contain small amounts of carbohydrates, proteins, vitamins, and minerals.

Chapter 3: Knowing your partners in fighting cholesterol

Nothing beats living a healthy lifestyle as a way to improve overall health. As you try to lower down your cholesterol, it is important to know your partners for better health because they can help you along the way. Read on.

What you should know about supplements

Americans spend billions worth of nutritional supplements. Some of them use it for nutritional insurance, while others see them as a shortcut to get all the vitamins and minerals they need without eating too much food.

When it comes to lowering cholesterol, experts found that some supplements may help raise your high-density lipoproteins (HDL) and lower total cholesterol. United States considers these supplements to be food products, instead of drugs. This is why they are not as strictly regulated as drugs, and only few studies show how certain pills can affect cholesterol, but every rule has an exception.

Essential vitamins and nutrients for lowering cholesterol

These are the vitamins and nutrients that you need to reduce total cholesterol:

> Niacin

Niacin is essential for development and growth. This B vitamin is involved in the creation of enzymes, which are natural compounds in the body that help run various processes, like digestion. You can get niacin from dairy products, grains, poultry, fish, and meat.

The Recommended Daily Allowance for adults is 14mg/NE for women, and 16mg/NE for men. A higher amount may be necessary to lower cholesterol levels.

> Calcium

You may have already heard countless times about how drinking milk every day can make your bones and teeth stronger. A 2003 study led by researchers from the University of Auckland in New Zealand reported that regularly taking calcium supplements may boost your HDL levels, and lower your LDLs.

> Dietary fiber

Many people do not know that there are two kinds of dietary fiber: insoluble and soluble. The former does not dissolve in your stomach, while the latter does. Experts say that eating foods rich in soluble fiber, like beans, veggies, fruits, and grains, can lower your cholesterol levels.

Soluble fiber mops up your cholesterol in the digestive tract before it reaches your bloodstream. You must take extra caution when considering taking soluble fiber rich foods or supplements because some people are allergic to psyllium. If you start having breathing trouble or feeling itchy, head to the nearest hospital or call an ambulance.

> Phytosterols

Phytosterols are natural substances found in plants that resemble cholesterol. Your body will absorb the phytosterols – which will not clog your arteries, by the way – and think it is cholesterol. Studies show that you must chug down at least 3,000mg of sterols every day to see a noticeable change in your total cholesterol levels. A tablespoon of sterol margarine contains 1,700mg of it, which means you only need to consume two tablespoons daily to meet the recommended amount.

Prescription medications and their side effects

Thanks to modern medicine, the number of deaths caused by heart attack declined. However, at present, it has not substantialy reduced the number of heart disease cases or heart attack related deaths. One way to make significant improvements is to eliminate what has been causing the many heart attacks, which is cholesterol.

Doctors are currently prescribing one or more of these medications to reduce cholesterol levels:

> Statin drugs

> Bile acid sequestrants

> Triglyceride inhibitors

People with high cholesterol, particularly those who have had a heart attack, may be given blood thinners like clopidogrel and aspirin. Blood thinners cannot lower cholesterol, but do reduce your risk of blood clotting.

Statins

Pravastatin, atorvastatin, fluvastatin, rosuvastatin, and simvastatin are examples of statin drugs. They work to:

> Reduce your LDLs

> Increase your HDLs

> Protect your arterial lining

> Reduce your plaque

> Lower your risk of heart attack

> Reduce your C-reactive protein, which is another risk factor for heart attack

> Lower your risk of a second heart attack (if you have already had one)

> Reduce your stroke risk

Statins are sold as single-ingredient or combo pills.

Common side effects: allergic rash, headache, fatigue, dizziness, upset stomach, low blood pressure, and abnormal results on liver enzyme test.

Less common side effects: Unusually low platelets, persistent unusual results on liver test, depression, muscle pain, muscle tenderness, memory loss, muscle loss, protein in urine.

You should not take a statin drug when you are taking antibiotics like erythromycin and clarithromycin, oral fungus medications like ketoconazole (and others whose names end in –azole), and protease inhibitors or drugs for HIV/AIDs. Be sure to tell your doctor what exactly you are currently taking.

Bile acid sequestrants

Bile acid sequestrants are natural compounds that gather bile acids in your intestines, and take them out through your feces. Bile acids are found in your gallbladder, where they are stored. If you have had your gallbladder removed, then your body will release bile acids straight into the digestive tract.

These acids allow your body to metabolize fat so you can absorb fatty acids, and convert them to cholesterol. You need to take the sequestrants before eating, so they are available when the gallbladder starts to produce bile acids. The cholesterol and triglycerides in your body will then be reduced.

Common side effects: loss of appetite, constipation, upset stomach, dizziness, headache, muscle and joint pains, and discolored teeth.

Less common side effects: vitamin deficiencies, reduced calcium absorption, reduced effectiveness of diuretics, painkillers, some antibiotics, some diabetes drugs, and some antifungal medications.

The Food and Drug Administration suggests that you start with small doses, stay well hydrated, and ask your doctor about whether you will need nutritional supplements.

Triglyceride inhibitors

These inhibitors work to reduce the amount of triglycerides produced by your liver. Triglycerides are fat that roams in your blood, and keeping the numbers low with the help of inhibitors will lower the creation of LDLs or the bad cholesterol. For unknown reasons, experts reported that these inhibitors can increase your HDL levels, as well.

Common side effects: blurred vision, itchy skin, allergic reaction, hives and rashes, fatigue, upset stomach, dizziness and headache, and muscle aches.

Less common side effects: gallstones, flu-like symptoms, lower potassium and white blood cell levels in the blood, muscle weakness, muscle tissue loss, and Raynaud's syndrom.

Medications that can raise cholesterol levels

Several common medications can help alleviate or cure certain conditions that they were designed to treat. However, they may also send your LDL or bad cholesterol levels up, and your HDL or good cholesterol down. These are:

> Birth control pills

Estrogen helps reduce total cholesterol levels, and increase the good cholesterol. However, taking higher doses of progestins will cause your good cholesterol levels to go down.

> Muscle builders

Anabolic androgenic steroids are taken by body builders to treat abnormally low testosterone levels. Steroid abuse, however, comes with several serious side effects like liver cancer, liver tumors, skin pigmentation (yellowish), hypertension, severe acne, kidney tumors, trembling, infertility, shrunken testicles, increased prostate cancer risk, and male-pattern baldness. It can also raise your LDLs, and reduce your HDLs.

> Hormone replacement therapy (HRT)

Women who are in the menopausal stage opt to undergo hormone replacement therapy. However, researchers have found a link between HRT and increased breast cancer risk. They have also disproved the belief that taking post-menopausal hormones will lower a woman's heart disease risk. For those who have been taking hormones, it is important to note that estrogen can increase a woman's HDL levels.

Every drug can be life-saving when it is prescribed for the condition it is designed to treat, as well as for those whose body can tolerate it. It is also crucial to understand that every drug has side effects. What works for one person might be dangerous for the other. The key is to minimize the risks and maximize the benefits.

Your Top 10 go-to websites for tips
Keep two things in mind when surfing the medical Web:

> Be cautious – Anyone can put up a website, so you are not always guaranteed credible information. Search for reputable websites, and avoid blogs and other sites that provide false promises.

> Read published studies that are less than five years old. Scientists discover new things once in a while, and what is be true today might get debunked in the next few years. Stay up-to-date with the latest findings from credible organizations or institutions.

Here are your top 10 go-to websites for cholesterol-lowering tips:

> The Cholesterol Low Down (by The American Heart Association)

www.cholesterollowdown.org

This website is part of the American Heart Association's national cholesterol education program. It aims to encourage everyone to see a doctor, check the cholesterol numbers, and come up with a long term plan for a healthy heart. This site has five pages that you can check: Getting Started, Get Active, Adjust Your Diet, Keep it Up, and Check Your Progress.

> Center for Drug Evaluation and Research www.fda.gov/cder/drug/default.htm

The CDER is a division of the FDA. Its website has valuable information and drug production evaluations. You will get millions of articles on everything linked to various medications, including those designed to help lower cholesterol levels.

> Center for Disease Control and Prevention www.cdc.gov/cholesterol

You can visit the CDC's website and search for a page dedicated to everything cholesterol, or simply click the link above. Here, you will find the latest news and press releases, as well as facts, prevention strategies, and statistics on certain issues like cholesterol.

> The Mayo Clinic www.mayohealth.org

The Mayo Clinic is a user-friendly website where people can easily gather information on certain medical issues, such as cholesterol. You can simply type cholesterol in the search box, and you will see hundreds of articles about it.

> National Cholesterol Education Program
www.nhlbi.nih.gov/guidelines/cholesterol/index.htm

In 1985, the National Heart, Lung, and Blood Institute launched this program with a goal of reducing death and illness caused by coronary heart disease in the United States. A part of their goal is to help Americans reduce their cholesterol levels. The website aims to raise awareness about high cholesterol as a serious risk factor for CHD, as well as the benefits of maintaining a healthy heart.

> The Food Allergy and Anaphylaxis Network www.foodallergy.org

The FAAN is a nonprofit organization that lets people join for as low as $30 a year. The members include families, dietitians, doctors, nurses, food manufacturers, and support groups in the United States, Europe, and Canada. This group offers educational information about food allergies, and provides coping strategies for people with allergic reactions to certain foods.

> The U.S. Department of Agriculture Nutrient Database
www.nal.usda.gov/fnic/cgi-bin/nut_search.pl

The USDA's Nutrient Database contains the most accurate nutrition chart. It helps measure cholesterol, vitamins, calories, and more. You can easily plan a low fat, low cholesterol diet with its chart. It provides nutrition data on thousands of foods, and breaks them down according to portions, sizes, and preparation methods.

> Food and Nutrition Information Center www.nal.usda.gov/fnic

The FNIC website is filled with nutrition facts, including links to information on how you can fight cholesterol. You will see recommended newsletters, magazines, books, and cookbooks that can teach you how to plan a cholesterol-lowering diet and reduce your heart disease risks.

> The Weight Control Information Network

www.niddk.nih.gov/health/nutrit/win.htm

Weight control is crucial in lowering cholesterol levels. The WIN website is one of the must-see sites because it gives you access to articles, audio-visual materials, and books connected to weight management. The website is managed by the National Institute of Diabetes and Digestive and Kidney Diseases, and the National Institutes of Health.

> The American Dietetic Association www.eatright.org

The ADA is the largest membership organization for nutrition professionals across the globe. Its website is packed with diet and food tips, research, guidelines, statistics, and policies that you can use. You will even see articles on how you can create a cholesterol-reducing meal plan. The best part of this website is where you can look for a nutrition professional in your area.

Here are the top 10 credible websites that you can check for health tips. However, you must know that the number of reliable sites can add up as the years pass. Stay up-to-date with the latest information and discoveries on cholesterol by visiting these websites regularly.

Chapter 4: Myth busters

You will find plenty of information available out there about the good and bad sides of cholesterol. However, not all of them are true. Some of them are only hear-says.

Unfortunately, many people continue to believe in things that have been disproven by science. How do you know which to believe? Below are the top 10 myth busters that anyone concerned about his or her health should know.

Myth #1: Most of the cholesterol comes from the food you eat

It is true that you get some cholesterol from the food you eat, but most of the ones floating in your bloodstream is made in your own body. The liver processes the fat, proteins, and carbohydrates that you eat to produce about a gram of cholesterol each day. Your body uses these homemade cholesterol to run various functions, like stimulating the brain to send messages back and forth.

Trouble may loom when you bring in more cholesterol from the food you eat. To maintain a healthy cholesterol level, the Dietary Guidelines for Americans recommends consuming no more than 300 milligrams of cholesterol a day from food.

Here is another surprise: The total amount of fat in your diet has now become more important than how much cholesterol you take in when determining your cholesterol level.

Myth #2: All fatty foods will raise your cholesterol levels

No. Why? All dietary fats are not alike. There are different kinds of fat, and they differ in terms of saturation, which is the amount of atoms sticking to the carbon atoms on fat molecules.

Saturated fatty acids, or saturated fat, raise the amount of fat in your blood. This includes the amount of LDLs that bring cholesterol into your arteries. Meanwhile, monounsaturated and polyunsaturated fatty acids may help reduce the number of fat in your blood and lower your bad cholesterol levels. The good fats can be found in high-fat plant-based foods, like avocados and nuts.

Do not get too excited yet. All fats relatively have high calories. In fact, they contain twice as many calories as carbohydrates and proteins. A high-calorie diet can increase your weight, and weight gain can raise your cholesterol levels. Do you see the connection now? Remember: not all dietary fats are bad, but taking in too much of the good ones can negatively affect your health.

Myth #3: Women are worry-free when it comes to cholesterol

The ladies tend to have lower cholesterol levels than men, from adolescence to middle age. A woman's body seems to be protected by the continuous flow of estrogen. Their cholesterol levels start to rise during menopause, where the production of estrogen gradually slows down.

Older women are more likely to have high cholesterol than men. However, a woman's blood vessels are more elastic, which means they are more likely to stay wide open than their counterpart's blood vessels. This amazing fact can protect older women against hypertension and blood clot.

Myth #4: Eat cholesterol-rich foods while you are young

Infants need fatty acids for growth and development. The American Academy of Pediatrics and American Heart Association recommend a meal plan with adequate fat for kids up to the age of two. By age 12, about seven out of ten

American children have fat deposits in their arteries. The AHA recommends getting a child older than two years old tested for cholesterol levels, particularly those with a family history of coronary artery disease.

Myth #5: Eat more fiber to lower cholesterol

Humans do not have the stomach to process insoluble fiber. One will need an extremely long gut and more than a stomach to digest it. When you consume insoluble fiber, it will travel through your intestines faster and reduce your risk of constipation, but will not lower your cholesterol levels.

Soluble fiber, on the other hand, can sop up cholesterol. Good examples include fruits, grains, and vegetables. When you take in plenty of soluble fiber, your cholesterol level will go down by about 10 percent or less.

Myth #6: Cholesterol is the sole culprit behind clogged arteries

Homocysteine, a type of amino acid, may equally be at fault. Your body produces this amino acid as a by-product of digested proteins. It circulates into your arteries, and can rough up the blood vessels. This creates ledges and chinks for cholesterol to cling onto. When cholesterol attaches to the arterial wall, it will lure more cholesterol particles, causing plaque build-up.

A diet packed with folate (a B vitamin) may help lower homocysteine levels, and reduce your risk of heart attack. Foods that are high in folic acid include green, leafy vegetables.

Myth #7: Heart attack is the only cholesterol-related health risk

Plaque build-up does not only occur in the coronary arteries. It may also develop in the arteries that send blood to the brain. The most common type of stroke, the cerebral thrombosis, happens when there is a blood clot in the cerebral blood vessel. It will block the pathway that sends blood and oxygen to the brain cells. The AHA reported that this form of stroke is most common in damaged arteries or those narrowed by plaque build-up.

Many people worry about the effects of elevated cholesterol levels on the coronary arteries. The truth is that high cholesterol levels may cause plaque build-up not only in the coronary blood vessels, but also to any other body part, even the penis. When there is a blocked blood vessel in the penis, it will definitely affect a man's ability to maintain erection.

Myth #8: Red meat contains more cholesterol than turkey and chicken

Red meat, including the lean ones, has more total fat than turkey or chicken, dark turkey or chicken (the legs and thighs) may bring in more cholesterol.

Myth #9: Cholesterol can never be too low

Believe it or not, having extremely low cholesterol level is also a huge problem. If your cholesterol level suddenly dives below 100mg/dL, then your doctor may not be happy with it if he or she finds out.

Hypocholesterolemia is the term used to describe very low cholesterol. It signals danger, such as malnutrition, liver cirrhosis, overactive thyroid glands, and certain cancer forms (like liver and colon cancer). It is no longer healthy when you have consistently low cholesterol levels. According to some researchers, it can trigger depression and suicidal tendencies as the brain may no longer produce enough serotonin – a brain chemical that makes you feel good.

Myth #10: Diet is the only way to regulate your cholesterol levels

You can only keep your cholesterol levels within the ideal range when you live a healthy lifestyle. It includes eating healthy, getting enough sleep, managing stress well, ditching vices, and exercising regularly. There are many factors that increase your risk of heart disease due to high cholesterol levels, and the only way to prevent this from happening is when you treat your mind and body well.

These are the top 10 cholesterol myths that have been busted by science. It is important to research thoroughly on things that you hear, especially if they are health-related. Aside from visiting the official websites of concerned government agencies and educational institutions, your doctor is one of the best persons to ask about your health. Never be afraid to set an appointment and ask every question in your head.

Chapter 5: Food is life

You have a reason to celebrate when your doctor finally breaks the good news: your cholesterol is now under control. People immediately think about unhealthy foods, sodas, and alcohol they hear the word "celebrate." Before you start worrying about putting your efforts to waste, there is a healthy and scrumptious way to celebrate your achievement. Read on.

Crunchy, but healthy

Healthy foods often lack the crunch, making you long for that crispy texture even more. Party favourites, such as tacos and potato chips, are crunchy but unhealthy. You can chew on crispy vegetable chips, home-baked whole wheat tortilla chips, crostini, and more.

Healthy appetizers

The good thing about party food is that it is filled with difficult-to-resist flavors. It is also full of fat and other unhealthy stuff. There is a way to indulge in fatty food, even if you are watching your cholesterol. The key is self-control. Here are your best options:

> Cheese

You can eat low- or non-fat cheese, or those soy-based cheeses. Low-fat ricotta, for example, can be extremely satisfying and guilt-free. Make sure to read the label for the total fat, cholesterol, and saturated fat content of each product you check. As much as possible, avoid Camembert, Roquefort, Brie, American-processed cheese, and cheddar as they contain more than 25 percent of the recommended daily allowance for saturated fat, and up to 10 percent of your cholesterol quota for the day.

Mozzarella and Feta are lower in both cholesterol and fat, and are the better choices. Who does not love mozzarella? Nearly everyone loves this stretchy cheese. You can use low-fat sour cream or yogurt, which are both palatable, to give that feeling of fat on the tongue.

> Nuts and olives

Olives and nuts are classic cocktail snacks that are heart-healthy. Studies show that these two snacks have been linked to reduced risk of heart disease. The mono- and polyunsaturated fat in these foods can help control cholesterol levels. With the wide variety of nuts available for human consumption, how do you know which of them are good to eat? Here are a few examples:

> Almonds

> Filberts

> Pecans

> Pistachios

> Walnuts

> Caviar

Caviar is a popular food choice for special occasions. These salted fish eggs are whole foods and are packed with nutrients. While most of its calories come from fat, caviar contains mostly poly- and monounsaturated fat. It is important to note, however, that this special occasion food is high in sodium, about 240mg per tablespoon. The good news is that you are not likely to eat a bowl-full of caviar, so there is no need to worry.

By now, you already know that the best way to control cholesterol is to learn the basics. These include knowing what cholesterol is, what it does, where it comes from, the health risks involved, why there are good and bad ones, and how you can regulate it to stay healthy. Lifestyle change is the overall solution to high cholesterol, and it is not as difficult as you think when you have the right information on hand.

ONE LAST THING...

If you enjoyed this book or found it useful I'd be very grateful if you'd post a short review here. Your support really does make a difference and I read all the reviews personally so I can get your feedback and make this book even better.

If you'd like to leave a review, then all you need to do is click the review link on this book's page.

Thanks again for your support!

This guide is not intended as and may not be construed as an alternative to or a substitute for professional business, mental counseling, therapy or medical services and advice

The authors, publishers, and distributors of this guide have made every effort to ensure the validity, accuracy, and timely nature of the information presented here However, no guarantee is made, neither direct nor implied, that the information in this guide or the techniques described herein are suitable for or applicable to any given individual person or group of persons, nor that any specific result will be achieved The authors, publishers, and distributors of this guide will be held harmless and without fault in all situations and causes arising from the use of this information by any person, with or without professional medical supervision The information contained in this book is for informational and entertainment purposes only It not intended as a professional advice or a recommendation to act

No part of this book may be reproduced or transmitted in any form whatsoever, electronic, or mechanical, including photocopying, recording, or by any informational storage or retrieval system without express permission from the author

© Copyright 2017, JNR Publishing

All rights reserved

Free bonus chapters of:

Foundations of the Gluten-free Diet

Rid yourself of celiac disease and more

Jessica Caplain

https://www.amazon.com/Foundations-Gluten-Free-Diet-yourself-disease-ebook/dp/B074PXM1TD/

Foundations of the Gluten-free Diet

Introduction to a Gluten-Free Lifestyle

What is Gluten?

Who Can Practice the Gluten-free Diet?

Why Going Gluten-Free Is the Best Decision You Could Make

Benefits of Gluten-Free Diets

What You Need to Know Before Starting a Gluten-Free Diet

Foods to Absolutely Avoid While On a Gluten-Free Diet

The Real Cost of a Gluten-Free Diet

Hard Truths about the Gluten Free Diet

Best Foods to Replace Wheat in Your Gluten-Free Diet

Eating Out While On a Gluten-free Diet

Gluten-Free Diet and Increased Energy

Energy Levels

How Does a Gluten-free Diet Affect Energy?

Improved Sleep

Gluten-free Diet and Improved Immune System

Common Colds and Flu

Allergies

Introduction to a Gluten-Free Lifestyle

The Gluten-free diet was initially meant for people who had Celiac disease. Celiac disease is characterized by a small intestine which is usually hypersensitive to gluten. This condition makes it difficult for food to be digested. Symptoms of this disease include abdominal bloating, anemia, skin rash, irregular menstrual periods and joint, muscle and bone pain.

Gluten-free diet is not meant for weight loss—though it is an incidental benefit in many instances. It is a form of treatment for people suffering from Celiac disease. It is also beneficial for people who may not have Celiac disease, but are still sensitive to gluten. There is no conventional medication for Celiac disease, so a 100% gluten-free diet is the only treatment available.

What is Gluten?

Gluten is a type of protein that is found in barley, rye, wheat and any other food product that is derived from them. Any diet that excludes these types of foods is touted as being gluten-free. So this means that you can live a gluten-free lifestyle and still eat healthy. Your diet will consist of animal protein, vegetables, fruits and dairy products.

You may be wondering whether a gluten-free diet means cutting out all grains? There are other grain alternatives that do not contain gluten, and can easily be substituted. These include millet, sorghum, corn, pea flour, potatoes, soy flour and amaranth. In as much as they do not contain gluten, these grains are also known as *cross-contact* grains. This is because they are grown where gluten produce is grown. So there is a chance that they come into contact with each other and hence traces of gluten can be found in foods that are meant to be gluten-free. For a person with Celiac disease, these small traces can cause inflammation of the intestines.

Who Can Practice the Gluten-free Diet?

As mentioned earlier, it is ideally meant for people who suffer from Celiac disease. This diet is also recommended if you have an allergic reaction to gluten. Another group of people who can benefit from a gluten-free diet are those who have allergic reactions to wheat. The extent of the reaction may vary, with some getting mild hives, and others going into anaphylactic shock.

The Gluten-free diet is quickly growing in popularity, and this book will give you all the information you need to know for a gluten-free diet. You will learn about the various advantages of going gluten-free such as improved digestive functions, increased energy and even weight loss.

You will also learn about what you need to know before you start this diet and any risks that may be involved. Furthermore, you will learn how to continue to live a gluten-free lifestyle even when you are not in control of your food, such as when eating out or even when traveling. Lastly, you will also learn about the best foods to replace gluten filled foods. Despite the fact you're not being able to eat certain foods, you would want to ensure that you still get the nutrients that are required for healthy living.

Why Going Gluten-Free Is the Best Decision You Could Make

Aside from those who have Celiac and are required to go gluten-free, why else would anyone willingly give up gluten products?

Benefits of Gluten-Free Diets

- If losing weight has been your struggle then you may be able to benefit from a gluten-free diet. Nutritionists agree that going gluten-free can help you lose otherwise stubborn fat. Gluten has a tendency to convert to fat, meaning if your diet is high in gluten, you will have trouble trying to lose weight. However, by cutting out gluten, you will be replacing it with healthy fruits and vegetables, which will give you the nutrition you need, while helping you stay healthy and be at your ideal weight. Gluten is also notorious for causing bloating, so once you cut it out of your diet, you will be surprised at how fast your tummy shrinks.

- Improved skin clarity and tone. Did you know that the reason you can't get rid of that pesky bout of acne could lie in your diet? Gluten can cause mild allergic reactions in some people, causing a rash or acne to break out. So if you have tried everything and nothing seems to work, it may be time to check your diet. Also, as a result of your increased intake of fruits and vegetables, your skin will be able to flush out toxins and it will have a natural glow.

- A diet high in gluten is responsible for most indigestion issues, bloating and fatigue. By cutting gluten from your diet, you will notice an almost immediate improvement in your digestion. If you suffer from indigestion or irregular bowel movements, then switching to a gluten-free diet will help give you comfort. Gluten clogs up your small intestines because it's a tad difficult to digest. As a result, most people suffer from chronic stomach pains.

Surprising Benefits of Going Gluten-Free

Aside from the major benefits that have been outlined above, here are some other things you may experience as a result of your newfound gluten-free lifestyle.

- Having worked out what you can and cannot eat in a gluten-free diet, you will feel the urge to fix up the rest of your diet by eliminating foods that may not be harmful but are not beneficial either. So now that you have eliminated gluten products, you suddenly realize that your body can do away with the artificial energy drinks you've been consuming daily. As a result of becoming conscious of what foods may or may not have gluten, you also become conscious of what you eat as a whole.

- You will enjoy cooking more. At first, it may seem like your options have been limited by eliminating all gluten products. However, this eventually makes you more creative in how you prepare your food. Surprisingly, you may even come up with your own original recipes. There are quite a number of gluten-free recipes that are available, and you can have a lot of fun replicating them or tweaking them to suit your fancy.

What You Need to Know Before Starting a Gluten-Free Diet

With all the hype surrounding gluten-free diets, and with more people joining this lifestyle, is it something that you would want to join as well? Before you do, here are several things you need to know.

It's a Need, a Want and Not Necessary

It does sound like a contradiction, doesn't it? But for people who suffer from Celiac, it is a required of them to avoid gluten as much as possible. This is especially important because there is no conventional medicine available that can treat Celiac completely.

There are also people who practice a gluten-free diet because they want to; perhaps as a result of their mild allergic reactions to wheat products.

Then there are those people who are doing it for its benefits such as weight loss and improved skin. In this case, a gluten-free diet may not be necessary, but you would still be free to practice it.

If You Suspect You Have Celiac, Consult With Your Doctor

You may have most of the symptoms of Celiac such as anemia, weight loss, stomach bloating and pain, but instead of just starting your gluten-free diet, it is advisable that you visit a doctor first.

BONUS FREE CHAPTER OF:

The Medical Self-Diagnosis Tool

Achieve better health by detecting and preventing illnesses, medical conditions and other disorders yourself!

Jessica Caplain

https://www.amazon.com/Medical-Self-Diagnosis-Tool-preventing-ebook/dp/B073Y5J6J7/

Introduction

The goal of this book is to teach the laymen practical ways to learn the skill of self-diagnosis without going overboard or it becoming dangerous. This is not meant to replace professional medical help. Far from it. This is just to aid the patient assess the situation as best as he can given his limited medical training and experiences and access to medical resources. Should the need arise, to make emergency decisions when called for. Of course it's preferable to always seek medical attention, but in the real world it may not always be possible due to lack of funds or simple unavailability of help.

Doctors absolutely hate patients who self-diagnose and self-medicate. Because they lack the training, they end up making things worse! I do not recommend this book as an alternative to seeking medical advice, rather this is meant to help take care of yourself until help arrives.

However not all conditions are serious enough to warrant a consultation with the doctor. You may do it too if you wish, but in some conditions it may be overkill such as a normal bacterial or viral infection such as cough and colds blown out of proportion to be mis-read as a serious medical event.

Know when you are out of your depth and seek a professional when in doubt. With that said, this book will give you tips and advice on how to best self-diagnose medical conditions and proper emergency responses.

In this book you will be taught the tools and proper mindset including approaches to correct self-diagnosis and treatment.

Identifying and Assessing Illnesses

Being able to Identify and deal with a medical condition doesn't come by chance. It needs insight and practical knowledge in the medical fields. With these, you can deal with various medical conditions before calling 911 or equivalent services. This skill is a potential life saver!

Understanding your health status

You are not immune to illness as you breathe, eat and drink. It is normal to experience a number of health problems, but knowing the specific causes and what to do can be help prevent things from getting worse. This is why you need knowledge in Self-Diagnosing health symptoms. You don't need to have an advanced degree in the medical sciences to be able to check on what is wrong and make decisions accordingly (within reason). With these basic skills, you can seek medical advice/treatment or manage it yourself.

Having a Medic Mentality

Some medical conditions are easy to detect while others are not because they are too complex for laymen or untrained personnel. But how do you know the difference? Some diagnoses however, are best done by professionals. For example, you may ignore the symptoms of a headache and take painkillers. So what do you do when it escalates? Hence a medic mentality.

Reacting to Medical Problems Sensibly

There are generally three ways people react to medical problems. These are:
- Dealing with it appropriately: Most people assess the cause of their health problem, seek professional advice and then deal with it.

- Having a 'stiff-upper-lip' attitude: These types are known as stoics as they act to the detriment of their health. They usually wait till others force them to seek medical treatment after their health symptoms have worsened.

- Worrying too much: Some people are very anxious about their health and therefore take every minor problem as a potentially serious medical condition. This pressures to them contact a health professional for assurance that the condition is not serious.

Dealing with your health conditions can be a little complicated. This can bring about making undue panic calls to health professionals which wastes their time better spent on other patients suffering from actual threatening health conditions. Think like a medic, and do this rather:

- Have patience: Don't make matters worse by getting too anxious. Most symptoms are not due to serious illnesses. However, seeking medical advice and getting reassurance is necessary to calm your mind.
- Buy time: Apart from medical emergencies like heart attacks and bleeding profusely, don't panic. You can do a general health check in the meantime.

Gaining basic skills in self diagnosis

With the right frame of mind, you can tackle health conditions like any other daily problem. For making prognosis follow these steps:

- Ask questions: You can make an early diagnosis by asking yourself the right questions about your health. This helps you size up the causes of your symptoms to decide whether they have a slight or serious impact on your health.

- Assess your body: Having a frequent physical check- ups help you notice signs of symptoms quickly. After noticing the symptoms, you can now make your next decision.

Identifying and Assessing Illnesses: The Basics

Looking at health behavior

According to researchers, there are differences in how people deal with their health problems based on diverse factors.

Feeling threatened: Many seek medical advice when the health condition is threatening or the other way around. For example, when the symptom is that of heart attack or HIV, professional advice is sought because they are scared enough.

Getting 'cues to action': With this, you may seek medical advice for physical symptoms after reading an article or watching a TV program on health. Yet again, the fear factor is motivating them to action.

Being on top of health concerns: You are confident in dealing with any symptom.

Perception about a medical condition: Your approach to a health condition can be affected by the environment or upbringing. This can make you ignore or act on the seriousness of a health risk. Medical conditions are best managed with self-awareness and objectivity.

Knowing how the body works

Knowing how the body is structured and works helps in self-diagnosing. This knowledge helps you to make sense of medical symptoms, because you know how the body system works. Let's begin with:

Free Sample Chapters:

Reverse Diabetes Fix Book

a diabetics solution for the best treatment plans to prevent & control pre-diabetes & the 2 types of diabetes & symptoms via exercise, diet, medications & alternative cures

Jessica Caplain

Get it here: https://www.amazon.com/dp/B076CP7K3F

Introduction
Types of Diabetes Mellitus
   Type I
   Type II
   Gestational
Possible Causes/Risk Factors
   Type I
   Type II
   Gestational
Signs and Symptoms
Complications
Diagnosis
   Type I and II
   Gestational
Treatment
   Type I
      Medications
      Exercise
      Diet
      Natural Home Remedies
   Type II Diabetes
      Medications
      Exercise
      Diet
      Natural Home Remedies
   Gestational Diabetes
      Medications
      Exercises
      Diet
      Natural Home Remedies
Conclusion

Introduction

Diabetes, also known as Diabetes Mellitus (DM) is an umbrella term for metabolic disorders that mostly spring from an issue in processing Insulin. Insulin is a pancreas-generated hormone that helps process glucose so the body can effectively transform it into energy, among other things.

Though DM is regarded as a metabolic disorder, it doesn't mean that only the endocrine and the gastrointestinal systems are affected. Remember, the body needs energy to function, and what better place to get this energy but from the GI system that supplies precious glucose to vital parts of the body, including the brain. This energy source (glucose) is used not only for energy production but also for growth and regeneration.

Types of Diabetes Mellitus

There are three main types of Diabetes. These are Type 1, Type 2, and Gestational Diabetes Mellitus.

Type I

Type 1 Diabetes is typically known as the Juvenile Type. As the name implies, young adults and children are the ones usually diagnosed with this condition. This is also known as the Insulin-dependent Type. Even if it's usually diagnosed during childhood, there are some instances that this disease has been discovered during people's adolescence or early adulthood.

People who have this condition usually cannot produce insulin with the help of the pancreas. Therefore, the body finds it hard to get some sugar from the blood. In turn, it's almost impossible to deliver energy from glucose to the different parts of the body.

Type II

Type 2 Diabetes also goes by names like Adult or Noninsulin-dependent Type. In this DM type, the pancreas may produce decreased amounts insulin for proper glucose processing. In some instances, the pancreas produces enough insulin but your body prevents your systems from using this. The adipose, liver, and contractile cells are just some of those that resist the effects of insulin in a person with DM.

This insulin restriction affects crucial functions like energy conversion and blood sugar regulation. The blood glucose levels skyrocket to levels beyond normal. At the same time, your energy stores become significantly lower. This is because most of the glycogen (a derivative of glucose) is stored in the blood and not in the muscles and liver where these should be. As a result, there's an imbalance that can significantly affect how your body heals itself, how it deals with stressful situations, and how it promotes overall balance inside your body.

Gestational

Pregnancy may lead to Gestational Diabetes, the third type. This is typically diagnosed during the third trimester. This condition develops mainly because of the placenta. The placenta contains various hormones that get released into the mother's bloodstream. This is not much of an issue during the first two trimesters mostly because of the size of the fetus and the number of systemic body functions that it has.

However, as the fetal development approaches the last trimester of pregnancy, the placenta secretes more hormones that are eventually brought to the mom's system. This sudden surge of hormones in the mother's body minimizes, if not disables, the blood sugar-regulating capabilities of the insulin.

Possible Causes/Risk Factors

The causes and risk factors for the Diabetes Mellitus types have distinct similarities. What makes each of them unique is the mechanism of how the problems eventually develop. It's important to know the possible causes and the factors that predispose you to have these conditions. Knowing these can help you avoid them or somewhat decrease their impact on your health in the long run.

Type I

The main cause of Type I Diabetes is technically unknown. However, one of the mechanisms that trigger this condition is the body's autoimmune reaction. When a person with Type I DM develops the condition, the body starts attacking the pancreas. The pancreas is the organ responsible for secreting juices that help in properly processing starch. When the pancreas breaks down the starch, the stomach absorbs this and distributes the nutrients to different parts of the body.

When the body starts attacking the pancreas, the organ has a hard time producing the juices. When this happens, the nutrients in starch and other food that you eat never get to different parts of the body where energy is needed. Instead, all the glucose and other body fuels stay in the bloodstream.

Some experts suspect genetics and even environmental factors (i.e., stress, food, alcohol, etc.) to be possible causes of Type I Diabetes as well. However, there is still no established research to support this claim – at least for now.

Here are some risk factors that can predispose you to have DM Type I:

*Location. People who live in colder countries seem to get this than those who live in warmer hemispheres.
*Race. Caucasians seem to get this type more than the other races.
*Family history.
*Presence of other autoimmune problems.
*Restrictive diet during younger age.
*Viral infections such as Mumps, Coxsackie, and German Measles.

Type II

Like Type I Diabetes, there is still no known established cause for Type II Diabetes. Experts speculate that this type also has external factors and heredity to blame. All they know is in Type II, the body just shuts the pancreas down. For some reason, the body seems to "think" that it's fed up with constant stimulation from the insulin that the pancreas produces. Because the body blocks off the insulin from this organ, blood sugar continues to shot up the more you eat or drink most foods or beverages with calories.

There are lots of risk factors that can cause you to end up with Type II DM. Some of these include the following:

*Obesity.

*Age. Older people get this condition more readily.

*Family history of DM Type II.

*Sedentary lifestyle.

*History of stroke or heart problems.

*History of Gestational Diabetes.

*Hypertension.

*History of PCOS (Polycystic Ovary Syndrome).

*High levels of triglycerides and/or low levels of "good cholesterol" (HDL).

Gestational

One of the main causes of this DM type is the inability of the pancreas to keep up with the body's demand for more insulin. As the third trimester approaches, the body will need more insulin because of the surge of hormones from the developing baby. Because the body can't keep up with the demands, too much glucose stays in the bloodstream, thus resulting in this DM type.

These are the factors that can increase the risk of having Gestational Diabetes:

*High blood sugar levels. This is known as Prediabetes. It's the blood sugar level between the normal values but a bit lower compared to the pregnant Diabetic.

*Family history of DM Type II.

*Age. Women older than 25 years old are highly susceptible to this condition.

*Obesity.

*History of unexplained miscarriage or stillbirth.

*History of PCOS or other hormonal problems.

*Race. Pacific Islanders, Hispanics, Asians, American Indians, and Africans are at higher risk.

*Hypertension.

Signs and Symptoms

The signs and symptoms of Diabetes Mellitus encompass most of the body systems. It's not much of a wonder because most of the body parts receive excessive amounts of glucose through the blood. Knowing these signs and symptoms of Diabetes Mellitus can help you determine if you need to address them through consultation and proper management. At the same time, this can help you act on the problem early so you can prevent serious complications in the future.

Increased incidences of infections. You can have more infections because the heightened blood sugar levels will eventually weaken your immune system. Also, other related problems like nerve problems and inefficient blood supply to different parts of your body make it difficult for your body to distribute the right nutrients needed for proper functioning and efficient regeneration of the body parts.

Slow-healing wounds. Again, high blood sugar levels are to blame for this. Because of excess glucose in your system, the blood has a hard time passing the right nutrients to the skin. In effect, the skin undergoes slower rates of inflammation, swelling, scab formation, and scar tissue formation. If left untreated, these wounds can also place you at risk of developing gangrene, bacterial infections, and fungal infections.

Dry skin. Because of high sugar levels in the blood, your skin tends to release moisture more readily. Because of this, you can see some brown and scaly patches in different parts of your body. This is typically known as Diabetic Dermopathy. Patches caused by this condition are often circular or round. They somewhat look like age spots. You can usually see them in front of your legs. Fortunately, these spots don't itch or hurt.

Extremely fatigued most of the time. Because of high levels of glucose in your blood, the blood has a harder time passing through the blood vessels. This slower rate of nutrient and oxygen distribution makes it harder for your cells to do their normal functions, in the same way as regeneration and repair become another set of issues as well. Conversely, hypoglycemic episodes (blood sugar levels that are lower than usual) limits the source of energy (glucose) that your body can have access to at the time.

Numbness or tingling in feet and hands. This is caused by damage to the nerves in your hands and feet. The sensation is usually accompanied by pain and weakness. This may also affect other parts of your body. When you have Diabetes, the body has a harder time getting nutrients that it needs because of inefficient blood flow. Because your nerves need blood more than most body parts, starvation will make their functions go haywire. Usually, patients with Diabetes describe the sensation as tingling, stabbing, or burning.

Sudden changes in vision. More glucose in the blood means thicker blood. When your blood is thicker, this encourages other surroundings fluids to pool in your eyes, among other parts. In turn, the lenses of your eyes will give you a hard time focusing on what you have to look at. This "swelling" of your eyes can be reversed if you address it as soon as possible.

Extreme thirst and frequent urination. Excessive thirst (polydipsia) is considered one of the classic signs and symptoms of DM. The increased levels of glucose in the blood force your kidneys to work double time to maintain the inner balance. However, there will come a time that they can no longer keep up with the demand. This will then encourage the body to excrete urine along with the excess sugar and fluids from different tissues. Because you urinate more often, you will eventually feel dehydrated, thus having the urge to drink more.

Unexplained weight loss. Weight changes happen because every time you get rid of excess glucose via urination, you tend to get rid of calories as well. At the same time, your condition can starve your cells by depriving them of valuable glucose supply. This, in effect, leads to constant hunger. The result is possible weight loss. This is especially applicable for people with Type I Diabetes.

Complications

Usually, complications from any type of Diabetes Mellitus develop rather slowly. If you let it go on without doing anything to manage your blood sugar levels, chances are you'll get most of these problems in the long run.

Heart problems. These include narrowing of the blood vessels, stroke, heart attack, regular chest pain, and coronary artery disease.

Hearing problems. This occurs because of poor blood supply to the nerves that are responsible for hearing.

Skin diseases. Because the skin is usually dry, untreated Diabetes can cause fungal and bacterial infections.

Foot problems. This is one of the most common complications in people with Diabetes. Aside from poor blood circulation to the feet, you may suffer from nerve damage. This, in turn, causes blisters and cuts to develop over time. As a result, poor wound healing and infections can take place.

Kidney diseases. Because glucose becomes constantly present in the kidneys even if it should not be, this causes damage to the blood vessels in these organs. This can cause the organs' filtering system to fail.

Eye problems. If left untreated, Diabetes can cause damaged retinas that can lead to blindness. This also increases your chances of developing other problems like glaucoma and cataract.

Pregnancy-related complications. For women with Gestational Diabetes, you may develop problems with your baby like excessive growth that will require C-section, low glucose levels, or even possible death before or during childbirth. As for the mother, complications like increased risks of Gestational Diabetes in future pregnancies and preeclampsia that can cause serious problems during or after childbirth.